KIDNEY DISEASE FOOD CHART

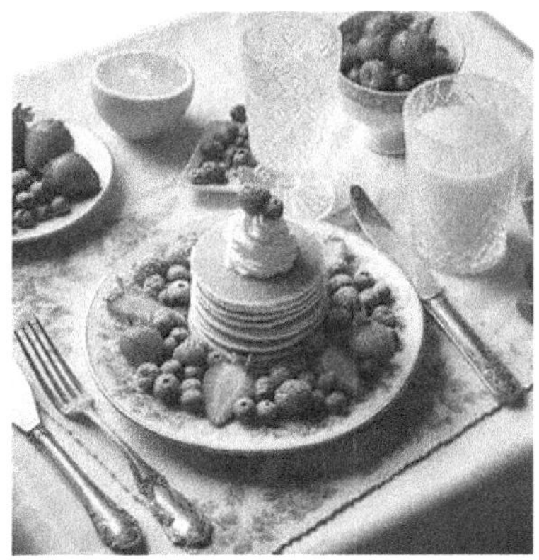

Explore a Palette of Low-Sodium, Low-Potassium, Low-Phosphorus, and Optimal Protein Foods with 300 Nutrient-Rich Recipes to Navigate and Enhance Your CKD Management

Tina Feldman

Table of Contents

Introduction 6

The Importance of Managing Diet for Kidney
Health 7

LOW PROTEIN FOOD CHART 10

Low-protein vegetables 10

Low protein fruits 13

Low-Protein Dairy Products 16

Nuts and Seeds 19

Low-Protein Sweeteners 23

Unsweetened Beverages 26

Herbs and Spices 30

Low-Protein Flours 33

Starches in Moderation 37

Fish and seafoods 44

Approved Kidney friendly Low sodium food
chart 51

Low-sodium yogurt 51

Nuts and seeds 54

Eggs 58

Lean meats and poultry 61

Beans and lentils 64

Whole grains 68

Vegetables 74

Unsweetened herbal tea 78

Sweeteners 81

Beverages 84

Baking and cooking ingredients 87

Protein Sources 90

kidney-friendly renal diet Meal Plan 93

Breakfast 93

Lunch 96

Dinner 99

Desserts 102

Snacks 104

Smoothies 107

Conclusion 110

Introduction

Kidney disease, also known as renal disease, refers to a condition where the kidneys' ability to function efficiently is compromised. The kidneys play a vital role in filtering waste products and excess fluids from the blood, regulating electrolyte balance, and maintaining overall fluid and blood pressure. When kidneys are impaired, they may struggle to perform these crucial functions, leading to a range of health complications.

One of the key aspects of managing kidney disease involves adopting a specialized diet known as the renal diet. This dietary approach aims to alleviate the strain on the kidneys by controlling the intake of certain nutrients, primarily sodium, potassium, phosphorus, and protein. The delicate balance of these elements is crucial for individuals with kidney disease to prevent the buildup of toxins and maintain optimal health.

Understanding the intricate relationship between kidney disease and diet is essential for those diagnosed with renal conditions. A well-planned renal diet can help manage symptoms, slow the progression of kidney disease, and improve overall quality of life. This dietary approach is often personalized based on the stage of kidney disease, individual health conditions, and specific nutritional needs.

In this context, it becomes imperative to explore and implement dietary strategies that not only support kidney function but also address nutritional requirements. Awareness of suitable food choices, portion control, and the avoidance of certain high-potassium, high-phosphorus, and high-sodium foods are integral components of a renal diet. Additionally, considering the impact of protein intake on kidney function is crucial, as excessive protein consumption can strain the kidneys.

As we delve into the intricacies of kidney disease and its connection to diet, it's important to acknowledge that nutritional management plays a pivotal role in empowering individuals to take an active role in their health. Working closely with healthcare professionals and registered dietitians can provide personalized guidance, ensuring that dietary choices align with both the individual's nutritional needs and the specific demands of managing kidney disease. Through a comprehensive understanding of the interplay between kidney health and nutrition, individuals can strive towards maintaining optimal well-being and enhancing their overall quality of life.

The Importance of Managing Diet for Kidney Health

Maintaining optimal kidney health is crucial for overall well-being, as the kidneys play a pivotal role in filtering waste products, regulating fluid balance, and managing electrolytes in the body. The impact of diet on kidney health cannot be overstated, and strategic dietary management is instrumental in preventing or slowing the progression of kidney disease. Here are key aspects highlighting the importance of managing diet for kidney health:

Controlling Blood Pressure:
A balanced diet, low in sodium and high in potassium, is essential for managing blood pressure. High blood pressure is a significant risk factor for kidney disease. By limiting sodium intake, individuals can help regulate blood pressure and reduce the strain on their kidneys.

Minimizing Protein Intake:
Protein is a crucial nutrient, but excessive consumption can burden the kidneys. For individuals with kidney disease, moderating protein intake is essential to prevent the accumulation of waste products in the blood. A tailored approach to protein intake, guided by healthcare professionals, ensures a balance that supports overall health.

Managing Fluid Balance:
Kidneys regulate fluid balance in the body. For individuals with kidney disease, monitoring fluid intake is vital to prevent fluid retention and maintain a healthy balance. Controlling the consumption of fluids, including water, can help prevent complications such as edema and high blood pressure.

Limiting Phosphorus Intake:
Phosphorus is a mineral that, in excess, can be harmful to individuals with kidney disease. Managing phosphorus intake is crucial to prevent bone and heart complications associated with elevated phosphorus levels. This often involves avoiding high-phosphorus foods and opting for kidney-friendly alternatives.

Addressing Potassium Levels:
Maintaining an appropriate balance of potassium is essential for heart and muscle function. Individuals with kidney disease need to monitor their potassium intake, as impaired kidney function can lead to potassium buildup. This involves making informed choices about potassium-rich foods.

Slowing the Progression of Kidney Disease:
Adhering to a renal diet can help slow the progression of kidney disease. By managing nutrient intake, individuals can reduce the workload on the kidneys and mitigate the risk of complications associated with advanced stages of kidney disease.

Enhancing Quality of Life:
A well-managed diet not only supports kidney health but also contributes to an improved overall quality of life. Individuals with kidney disease may experience increased energy levels, better weight management, and a reduced risk of complications, enhancing their daily well-being.

Individualized Nutrition Plans:
Each person's nutritional needs are unique. Collaborating with healthcare professionals, including registered dietitians, ensures the development of personalized nutrition plans tailored to specific kidney health requirements, stage of kidney disease, and individual health goals.

LOW PROTEIN FOOD CHART

Low-protein vegetables

Cucumber:
Serving Size: 1 cup (104g)
Calories: 16
Protein: 0.8g
Cholesterol: 0mg

Cauliflower:
Serving Size: 1 cup (100g)
Calories: 25
Protein: 2g
Cholesterol: 0mg

Zucchini:
Serving Size: 1 cup (180g)
Calories: 20
Protein: 1.4g
Cholesterol: 0mg

Bell Peppers:
Serving Size: 1 cup (149g)
Calories: 46

Protein: 1.5g
Cholesterol: 0mg

Eggplant:
Serving Size: 1 cup (82g)
Calories: 20
Protein: 0.8g
Cholesterol: 0mg

Broccoli:
Serving Size: 1 cup (156g)
Calories: 55
Protein: 4.2g
Cholesterol: 0mg

Spinach:
Serving Size: 1 cup (30g)
Calories: 7
Protein: 0.9g
Cholesterol: 0mg

Cabbage:
Serving Size: 1 cup (89g)
Calories: 22
Protein: 1.1g
Cholesterol: 0mg

Green Beans:
Serving Size: 1 cup (125g)
Calories: 31
Protein: 2g
Cholesterol: 0mg

Asparagus:
Serving Size: 1 cup (134g)
Calories: 27
Protein: 2.9g
Cholesterol: 0mg

Mushrooms:
Serving Size: 1 cup (96g)
Calories: 21
Protein: 3g
Cholesterol: 0mg

Brussels Sprouts:
Serving Size: 1 cup (88g)
Calories: 38
Protein: 3g
Cholesterol: 0mg

Radishes:
Serving Size: 1 cup (116g)
Calories: 19
Protein: 0.8g
Cholesterol: 0mg

Celery:
Serving Size: 1 cup (101g)
Calories: 16
Protein: 0.8g
Cholesterol: 0mg

Cabbage (Napa):
Serving Size: 1 cup (100g)
Calories: 12

Protein: 1g
Cholesterol: 0mg

Low protein fruits

Strawberries:
Serving Size: 1 cup (144g)
Calories: 49
Protein: 1g
Cholesterol: 0mg

Blueberries:
Serving Size: 1 cup (148g)
Calories: 84
Protein: 1g
Cholesterol: 0mg

Peaches:
Serving Size: 1 medium peach (150g)
Calories: 58
Protein: 1.4g
Cholesterol: 0mg

Raspberries:
Serving Size: 1 cup (123g)
Calories: 64
Protein: 1.5g
Cholesterol: 0mg

Cranberries (fresh):
Serving Size: 1 cup (100g)
Calories: 46
Protein: 0.4g

Cholesterol: 0mg

Watermelon:
Serving Size: 1 cup (152g)
Calories: 46
Protein: 0.9g
Cholesterol: 0mg

Papaya:
Serving Size: 1 cup (140g)
Calories: 55
Protein: 0.9g
Cholesterol: 0mg

Apricots:
Serving Size: 1 medium apricot (35g)
Calories: 17
Protein: 0.5g
Cholesterol: 0mg

Plums:
Serving Size: 2 medium plums (151g)
Calories: 70
Protein: 0.7g
Cholesterol: 0mg

Kiwi:
Serving Size: 1 medium kiwi (100g)
Calories: 61
Protein: 1.1g
Cholesterol: 0mg

Cantaloupe:
Serving Size: 1 cup (160g)
Calories: 54
Protein: 1.3g
Cholesterol: 0mg

Grapes:
Serving Size: 1 cup (151g)
Calories: 104
Protein: 1.1g
Cholesterol: 0mg

Apples:
Serving Size: 1 medium apple (182g)
Calories: 95
Protein: 0.5g
Cholesterol: 0mg

Mango:
Serving Size: 1 cup (165g)
Calories: 99
Protein: 1.4g
Cholesterol: 0mg

Oranges:
Serving Size: 1 medium orange (131g)
Calories: 62
Protein: 1.2g
Cholesterol: 0mg

Low-Protein Dairy Products

Skim Milk:
Serving Size: 1 cup (240ml)
Calories: 80
Protein: 8g
Cholesterol: 5mg
Note: Skim milk has lower fat content and is a good source of calcium.

Almond Milk (Unsweetened):
Serving Size: 1 cup (240ml)
Calories: 30
Protein: 1g
Cholesterol: 0mg
Note: Almond milk is a non-dairy alternative suitable for those with lactose intolerance.

Cottage Cheese (Low-Fat):
Serving Size: 1 cup (226g)
Calories: 206
Protein: 28g
Cholesterol: 11mg
Note: Choose low-fat options to reduce saturated fat intake.

Greek Yogurt (Low-Fat):
Serving Size: 1 cup (227g)
Calories: 146
Protein: 23g
Cholesterol: 28mg
Note: Greek yogurt is often higher in protein, so moderation is key.

Soy Milk (Unsweetened):
Serving Size: 1 cup (240ml)
Calories: 80
Protein: 7g
Cholesterol: 0mg
Note: Soy milk is a plant-based alternative with less protein than cow's milk.

Ricotta Cheese (Part-Skim):
Serving Size: 1 cup (248g)
Calories: 339
Protein: 28g
Cholesterol: 88mg
Note: Part-skim options contain less fat.

Coconut Milk (Unsweetened):
Serving Size: 1 cup (240ml)
Calories: 50
Protein: 0g
Cholesterol: 0mg
Note: Coconut milk is a dairy-free option with no protein.

Mozzarella Cheese (Part-Skim):
Serving Size: 1 ounce (28g)
Calories: 71
Protein: 6g
Cholesterol: 18mg
Note: Part-skim mozzarella is lower in fat.

Non-Dairy Yogurt (Low-Protein):
Serving Size: 1 cup (240ml)
Calories: Varies (check the label)

Protein: Varies (check the label)
Cholesterol: Varies (check the label)
Note: Choose non-dairy yogurt with lower protein content.

Buttermilk (Low-Fat):
Serving Size: 1 cup (245g)
Calories: 98
Protein: 8g
Cholesterol: 12mg
Note: Low-fat buttermilk can be a lower-protein alternative.

Swiss Cheese (Reduced-Fat):
Serving Size: 1 slice (28g)
Calories: 50
Protein: 5g
Cholesterol: 12mg
Note: Opt for reduced-fat versions of cheese.

Feta Cheese (Reduced-Fat):
Serving Size: 1 ounce (28g)
Calories: 36
Protein: 4g
Cholesterol: 13mg
Note: Reduced-fat feta is a lower-protein option.

Provolone Cheese (Reduced-Fat):
Serving Size: 1 slice (28g)
Calories: 50
Protein: 5g
Cholesterol: 12mg

Note: Choose reduced-fat options for lower protein content.

Sour Cream (Reduced-Fat):
Serving Size: 2 tablespoons (30g)
Calories: 40
Protein: 1g
Cholesterol: 10mg
Note: Opt for reduced-fat sour cream for lower protein and fat content.

Whipped Cream (Light):
Serving Size: 2 tablespoons (30g)
Calories: 15
Protein: 0g
Cholesterol: 0mg
Note: Light whipped cream is a low-protein topping option.

Nuts and Seeds

Almonds (Raw):
Serving Size: 1 ounce (28g)
Calories: 160
Protein: 6g
Cholesterol: 0mg
Note: Choose raw almonds without added salt for a lower-protein option.

Peanuts (Dry-Roasted):
Serving Size: 1 ounce (28g)
Calories: 166
Protein: 7g

Cholesterol: 0mg
Note: Opt for dry-roasted peanuts without added salt for reduced protein content.

Sunflower Seeds (Hulled):
Serving Size: 1 ounce (28g)
Calories: 163
Protein: 6g
Cholesterol: 0mg
Note: Hulled sunflower seeds are a lower-protein option.

Pumpkin Seeds (Pepitas):
Serving Size: 1 ounce (28g)
Calories: 151
Protein: 7g
Cholesterol: 0mg
Note: Pumpkin seeds are a good source of nutrients with moderate protein content.

Cashews (Raw):
Serving Size: 1 ounce (28g)
Calories: 157
Protein: 5g
Cholesterol: 0mg
Note: Choose raw cashews without added salt for a lower-protein option.

Walnuts (Raw):
Serving Size: 1 ounce (28g)
Calories: 185
Protein: 4g
Cholesterol: 0mg

Note: Raw walnuts are a good source of omega-3 fatty acids with moderate protein content.

Hazelnuts (Raw):
Serving Size: 1 ounce (28g)
Calories: 178
Protein: 4g
Cholesterol: 0mg
Note: Choose raw hazelnuts for a lower-protein option.

Macadamia Nuts (Raw):
Serving Size: 1 ounce (28g)
Calories: 204
Protein: 2g
Cholesterol: 0mg
Note: Macadamia nuts have a higher fat content and lower protein.

Pecans (Raw):
Serving Size: 1 ounce (28g)
Calories: 196
Protein: 3g
Cholesterol: 0mg
Note: Raw pecans are a lower-protein nut option.

Chia Seeds:
Serving Size: 1 ounce (28g)
Calories: 138
Protein: 4g
Cholesterol: 0mg
Note: Chia seeds are rich in omega-3 fatty acids and fiber.

Flaxseeds:
Serving Size: 1 ounce (28g)
Calories: 150
Protein: 5g
Cholesterol: 0mg
Note: Ground flaxseeds are a good source of omega-3 fatty acids.

Hemp Seeds:
Serving Size: 1 ounce (28g)
Calories: 154
Protein: 9g
Cholesterol: 0mg
Note: Hemp seeds are a complete protein source.

Brazil Nuts (Raw):
Serving Size: 1 ounce (28g)
Calories: 186
Protein: 4g
Cholesterol: 0mg
Note: Brazil nuts are high in selenium and lower in protein.

Sesame Seeds:
Serving Size: 1 ounce (28g)
Calories: 160
Protein: 5g
Cholesterol: 0mg
Note: Sesame seeds are a versatile, lower-protein option.

Pistachios (Raw):
Serving Size: 1 ounce (28g)

Calories: 156
Protein: 6g
Cholesterol: 0mg
Note: Raw pistachios are a tasty nut with moderate protein content.

Low-Protein Sweeteners

Stevia (Pure Extract):
Serving Size: 1 packet (1g)
Calories: 0
Protein: 0g
Cholesterol: 0mg
Note: Stevia is a natural, calorie-free sweetener.

Monk Fruit Extract:
Serving Size: 1 teaspoon (1.7g)
Calories: 0
Protein: 0g
Cholesterol: 0mg
Note: Monk fruit extract is a natural, zero-calorie sweetener.

Erythritol:
Serving Size: 1 teaspoon (4g)
Calories: 0
Protein: 0g
Cholesterol: 0mg
Note: Erythritol is a sugar alcohol with zero calories.

Xylitol:
Serving Size: 1 teaspoon (4g)
Calories: 10
Protein: 0g

Cholesterol: 0mg
Note: Xylitol is a sugar alcohol with a low glycemic
index.

Aspartame (Equal):
Serving Size: 1 packet (1.8g)
Calories: 4
Protein: 0g
Cholesterol: 0mg
Note: Aspartame is a low-calorie sweetener.

Sucralose (Splenda):
Serving Size: 1 packet (1g)
Calories: 3
Protein: 0g
Cholesterol: 0mg
Note: Sucralose is a non-nutritive sweetener.

Saccharin (Sweet'N Low):
Serving Size: 1 packet (1.7g)
Calories: 4
Protein: 0g
Cholesterol: 0mg
Note: Saccharin is a non-nutritive sweetener.

Acesulfame Potassium (Sunett):
Serving Size: 1 packet (1g)
Calories: 0
Protein: 0g
Cholesterol: 0mg
Note: Acesulfame potassium is a calorie-free
sweetener.

Agave Nectar:
Serving Size: 1 tablespoon (21g)
Calories: 60
Protein: 0g
Cholesterol: 0mg
Note: Agave nectar is a natural sweetener with a lower glycemic index.

Coconut Sugar:
Serving Size: 1 teaspoon (4g)
Calories: 15
Protein: 0g
Cholesterol: 0mg
Note: Coconut sugar is a natural sweetener with a distinct flavor.

Maple Syrup (Pure):
Serving Size: 1 tablespoon (20g)
Calories: 52
Protein: 0g
Cholesterol: 0mg
Note: Choose pure maple syrup without added sugars.

Date Sugar:
Serving Size: 1 teaspoon (4g)
Calories: 15
Protein: 0g
Cholesterol: 0mg
Note: Date sugar is made from dried dates and adds natural sweetness.

Honey (Pure):
Serving Size: 1 tablespoon (21g)
Calories: 64
Protein: 0.1g
Cholesterol: 0mg
Note: Choose pure honey without added sugars.

Molasses (Blackstrap):
Serving Size: 1 tablespoon (20g)
Calories: 47
Protein: 0.7g
Cholesterol: 0mg
Note: Blackstrap molasses is rich in minerals and has a robust flavor.

Brown Rice Syrup:
Serving Size: 1 tablespoon (20g)
Calories: 55
Protein: 0.1g
Cholesterol: 0mg
Note: Brown rice syrup is a less refined sweetener with a mild taste.

Unsweetened Beverages

Water:
Serving Size: 8 fl oz (240ml)
Calories: 0
Protein: 0g
Cholesterol: 0mg
Note: Water is a calorie-free and protein-free option.

Herbal Tea (Unsweetened):
Serving Size: 8 fl oz (240ml)

Calories: 0
Protein: 0g
Cholesterol: 0mg
Note: Herbal teas, without added sweeteners, are a low-calorie option.

Black Coffee (Unsweetened):
Serving Size: 8 fl oz (240ml)
Calories: 2
Protein: 0g
Cholesterol: 0mg
Note: Black coffee is low in calories and protein.

Green Tea (Unsweetened):
Serving Size: 8 fl oz (240ml)
Calories: 0
Protein: 0g
Cholesterol: 0mg
Note: Unsweetened green tea is a low-calorie and low-protein option.

Almond Milk (Unsweetened):
Serving Size: 8 fl oz (240ml)
Calories: 30
Protein: 1g
Cholesterol: 0mg
Note: Almond milk is a dairy-free alternative with lower protein content.

Coconut Water:
Serving Size: 8 fl oz (240ml)
Calories: 46
Protein: 2g

Cholesterol: 0mg
Note: Coconut water is a natural, hydrating option.

Sparkling Water (Unsweetened):
Serving Size: 8 fl oz (240ml)
Calories: 0
Protein: 0g
Cholesterol: 0mg
Note: Sparkling water without added sweeteners is a refreshing, calorie-free choice.

Unsweetened Soy Milk:
Serving Size: 8 fl oz (240ml)
Calories: 80
Protein: 7g
Cholesterol: 0mg
Note: Unsweetened soy milk is a plant-based alternative with lower protein.

Clear Broth (Chicken or Vegetable):
Serving Size: 8 fl oz (240ml)
Calories: 10
Protein: 1g
Cholesterol: 0mg
Note: Clear broth is a low-calorie, low-protein option.

Unsweetened Rice Milk:
Serving Size: 8 fl oz (240ml)
Calories: 70
Protein: 0g
Cholesterol: 0mg

Note: Unsweetened rice milk is another dairy-free alternative.

Lemonade (Freshly Squeezed, No Sugar Added):
Serving Size: 8 fl oz (240ml)
Calories: 7
Protein: 0.1g
Cholesterol: 0mg
Note: Freshly squeezed lemonade without added sugar is a low-calorie choice.

Tomato Juice (Low-Sodium):
Serving Size: 8 fl oz (240ml)
Calories: 41
Protein: 2g
Cholesterol: 0mg
Note: Low-sodium tomato juice is a lower-protein option.

Hibiscus Tea (Unsweetened):
Serving Size: 8 fl oz (240ml)
Calories: 0
Protein: 0g
Cholesterol: 0mg
Note: Hibiscus tea is a caffeine-free and low-calorie beverage.

Vegetable Juice (Low-Sodium):
Serving Size: 8 fl oz (240ml)
Calories: 50
Protein: 2g
Cholesterol: 0mg

Note: Low-sodium vegetable juice is a source of vitamins with moderate protein.

Iced Peppermint Tea (Unsweetened):
Serving Size: 8 fl oz (240ml)
Calories: 0
Protein: 0g
Cholesterol: 0mg
Note: Unsweetened peppermint tea is a refreshing, calorie-free option.

Herbs and Spices

Basil:
Serving Size: 1 tablespoon (2g)
Calories: 1
Protein: 0.1g
Cholesterol: 0mg

Thyme:
Serving Size: 1 teaspoon (1g)
Calories: 3
Protein: 0.1g
Cholesterol: 0mg

Rosemary:
Serving Size: 1 teaspoon (1g)
Calories: 2
Protein: 0.1g
Cholesterol: 0mg

Oregano:
Serving Size: 1 teaspoon (1g)
Calories: 3
Protein: 0.1g
Cholesterol: 0mg

Cilantro (Coriander):
Serving Size: 1 tablespoon (4g)
Calories: 0
Protein: 0g
Cholesterol: 0mg

Parsley:
Serving Size: 1 tablespoon (3g)
Calories: 1
Protein: 0.1g
Cholesterol: 0mg

Dill Weed:
Serving Size: 1 teaspoon (1g)
Calories: 3
Protein: 0.1g
Cholesterol: 0mg

Chives:
Serving Size: 1 tablespoon (3g)
Calories: 1
Protein: 0.1g
Cholesterol: 0mg

Garlic Powder:
Serving Size: 1 teaspoon (3g)
Calories: 10

Protein: 0.4g
Cholesterol: 0mg

Ginger (Ground):
Serving Size: 1 teaspoon (2g)
Calories: 5
Protein: 0.1g
Cholesterol: 0mg

Turmeric (Ground):
Serving Size: 1 teaspoon (2g)
Calories: 8
Protein: 0.2g
Cholesterol: 0mg

Cumin (Ground):
Serving Size: 1 teaspoon (2g)
Calories: 8
Protein: 0.3g
Cholesterol: 0mg

Cayenne Pepper:
Serving Size: 1 teaspoon (2g)
Calories: 6
Protein: 0.3g
Cholesterol: 0mg

Paprika:
Serving Size: 1 teaspoon (2g)
Calories: 6
Protein: 0.2g
Cholesterol: 0mg

Coriander (Ground):
Serving Size: 1 teaspoon (2g)
Calories: 6
Protein: 0.3g
Cholesterol: 0mg

Low-Protein Flours

Almond Flour:
Serving Size: 1/4 cup (28g)
Calories: 160
Protein: 6g
Cholesterol: 0mg
Note: Almond flour is relatively high in protein compared to other flours but can be used in moderation.

Coconut Flour:
Serving Size: 1/4 cup (28g)
Calories: 120
Protein: 4g
Cholesterol: 0mg
Note: Coconut flour is a gluten-free option with moderate protein.

Rice Flour:
Serving Size: 1/4 cup (30g)
Calories: 110
Protein: 2g
Cholesterol: 0mg
Note: Rice flour is a versatile, gluten-free option.

Quinoa Flour:
Serving Size: 1/4 cup (30g)

Calories: 110
Protein: 4g
Cholesterol: 0mg
Note: Quinoa flour is higher in protein but can be used in moderation.

Chickpea Flour (Besan):
Serving Size: 1/4 cup (30g)
Calories: 110
Protein: 6g
Cholesterol: 0mg
Note: Chickpea flour is higher in protein and may be suitable in limited amounts.

Buckwheat Flour:
Serving Size: 1/4 cup (30g)
Calories: 110
Protein: 4g
Cholesterol: 0mg
Note: Buckwheat flour is gluten-free and has moderate protein.

Sorghum Flour:
Serving Size: 1/4 cup (30g)
Calories: 110
Protein: 4g
Cholesterol: 0mg
Note: Sorghum flour is gluten-free and lower in protein.

Tapioca Flour:
Serving Size: 1/4 cup (30g)
Calories: 100

Protein: 0g
Cholesterol: 0mg
Note: Tapioca flour is often used as a thickening agent and is low in protein.

Arrowroot Flour:
Serving Size: 1/4 cup (30g)
Calories: 110
Protein: 0g
Cholesterol: 0mg
Note: Arrowroot flour is a gluten-free option with no protein.

Millet Flour:
Serving Size: 1/4 cup (30g)
Calories: 100
Protein: 3g
Cholesterol: 0mg
Note: Millet flour is a gluten-free option with moderate protein.

Oat Flour:
Serving Size: 1/4 cup (30g)
Calories: 110
Protein: 4g
Cholesterol: 0mg
Note: Oat flour can be a good option if tolerated in moderation.

Cassava Flour:
Serving Size: 1/4 cup (30g)
Calories: 100
Protein: 0g

Cholesterol: 0mg
Note: Cassava flour is grain-free and low in protein.

Soy Flour:
Serving Size: 1/4 cup (30g)
Calories: 120
Protein: 12g
Cholesterol: 0mg
Note: Soy flour is relatively high in protein and should be used in moderation.

Potato Flour:
Serving Size: 1/4 cup (30g)
Calories: 110
Protein: 2g
Cholesterol: 0mg
Note: Potato flour is a gluten-free option with lower protein.

Hemp Flour:
Serving Size: 1/4 cup (30g)
Calories: 120
Protein: 12g
Cholesterol: 0mg
Note: Hemp flour is higher in protein and should be used in moderation.

White Potatoes (Boiled):
Serving Size: 1 medium potato (150g)
Calories: 110
Protein: 2g
Cholesterol: 0mg
Note: Rich in carbohydrates, potatoes can be a part of a kidney-friendly diet in moderation.

Sweet Potatoes (Baked):
Serving Size: 1 medium sweet potato (114g)
Calories: 103
Protein: 2g
Cholesterol: 0mg
Note: Sweet potatoes are a good source of vitamins and minerals.

White Rice (Cooked):
Serving Size: 1 cup (195g)
Calories: 218
Protein: 4g
Cholesterol: 0mg
Note: White rice is a low-phosphorus option when consumed in moderation.

Brown Rice (Cooked):
Serving Size: 1 cup (195g)
Calories: 215
Protein: 5g
Cholesterol: 0mg
Note: Brown rice is a whole grain with added fiber.

Quinoa (Cooked):
Serving Size: 1 cup (185g)
Calories: 222
Protein: 8g
Cholesterol: 0mg
Note: Quinoa is a complete protein and a good source
of fiber.

Barley (Cooked):
Serving Size: 1 cup (157g)
Calories: 193
Protein: 4g
Cholesterol: 0mg
Note: Barley is a high-fiber grain.

Couscous (Cooked):
Serving Size: 1 cup (157g)
Calories: 176
Protein: 6g
Cholesterol: 0mg
Note: Couscous is a quick-cooking grain.

Oats (Cooked):
Serving Size: 1 cup (234g)
Calories: 166
Protein: 6g
Cholesterol: 0mg
Note: Oats are a good source of soluble fiber.

Whole Wheat Pasta (Cooked):
Serving Size: 1 cup (140g)
Calories: 174
Protein: 7g

Cholesterol: 0mg
Note: Choose whole wheat for added fiber.

Butternut Squash (Baked):
Serving Size: 1 cup cubes (205g)
Calories: 82
Protein: 2g
Cholesterol: 0mg
Note: Butternut squash is a nutrient-dense starchy vegetable.

Corn (Boiled):
Serving Size: 1 cup kernels (154g)
Calories: 132
Protein: 4g
Cholesterol: 0mg
Note: Corn can be included in moderation.

Pumpkin (Baked):
Serving Size: 1 cup cubes (116g)
Calories: 30
Protein: 1g
Cholesterol: 0mg
Note: Pumpkin is low in calories and can be used in various dishes.

Acorn Squash (Baked):
Serving Size: 1 cup cubes (205g)
Calories: 115
Protein: 1g
Cholesterol: 0mg
Note: Acorn squash is a winter squash with a sweet flavor.

Plantains (Boiled):
Serving Size: 1 medium plantain (179g)
Calories: 218
Protein: 1g
Cholesterol: 0mg
Note: Plantains can be included in moderation.

Spaghetti Squash (Cooked):
Serving Size: 1 cup strands (155g)
Calories: 42
Protein: 1g
Cholesterol: 0mg
Note: Spaghetti squash is a low-calorie alternative to traditional pasta.

Olive Oil (Extra Virgin):
Serving Size: 1 tablespoon (14g)
Calories: 119
Protein: 0g
Cholesterol: 0mg
Note: A heart-healthy option with monounsaturated fats.

Canola Oil:
Serving Size: 1 tablespoon (14g)
Calories: 124
Protein: 0g
Cholesterol: 0mg
Note: Low in saturated fats, suitable for cooking.

Avocado Oil:
Serving Size: 1 tablespoon (14g)
Calories: 124

Protein: 0g
Cholesterol: 0mg
Note: Rich in monounsaturated fats and suitable for high-heat cooking.

Coconut Oil:
Serving Size: 1 tablespoon (13.6g)
Calories: 120
Protein: 0g
Cholesterol: 0mg
Note: High in saturated fats, use in moderation.

Flaxseed Oil:
Serving Size: 1 tablespoon (14g)
Calories: 120
Protein: 0g
Cholesterol: 0mg
Note: A source of omega-3 fatty acids, avoid heating.

Walnut Oil:
Serving Size: 1 tablespoon (14g)
Calories: 120
Protein: 0g
Cholesterol: 0mg
Note: Contains omega-3 fatty acids, suitable for salads.

Sesame Oil:
Serving Size: 1 tablespoon (13.6g)
Calories: 120
Protein: 0g
Cholesterol: 0mg
Note: Adds a distinct flavor, use in moderation.

Grapeseed Oil:
Serving Size: 1 tablespoon (14g)
Calories: 120
Protein: 0g
Cholesterol: 0mg
Note: Suitable for high-heat cooking, neutral flavor.

Peanut Oil:
Serving Size: 1 tablespoon (14g)
Calories: 120
Protein: 0g
Cholesterol: 0mg
Note: Ideal for frying, use in moderation.

Sunflower Oil:
Serving Size: 1 tablespoon (13.6g)
Calories: 120
Protein: 0g
Cholesterol: 0mg
Note: A neutral oil, suitable for cooking.

Corn Oil:
Serving Size: 1 tablespoon (13.6g)
Calories: 120
Protein: 0g
Cholesterol: 0mg
Note: A versatile cooking oil, use in moderation.

Safflower Oil:
Serving Size: 1 tablespoon (13.6g)
Calories: 120
Protein: 0g

Cholesterol: 0mg
Note: Suitable for cooking at high temperatures.

MCT Oil (Medium-Chain Triglycerides):
Serving Size: 1 tablespoon (14g)
Calories: 100
Protein: 0g
Cholesterol: 0mg
Note: Easily digestible, used for energy, but consult a healthcare professional.

Butter (Unsalted):
Serving Size: 1 tablespoon (14g)
Calories: 102
Protein: 0.1g
Cholesterol: 31mg
Note: High in saturated fats, use in moderation.

Lard:
Serving Size: 1 tablespoon (12.8g)
Calories: 115
Protein: 0.1g
Cholesterol: 11mg
Note: High in saturated fats, use sparingly.

Fish and seafoods

Salmon (Wild-Caught, Cooked):
Serving Size: 3 ounces (85g)
Calories: 155
Protein: 22g
Cholesterol: 63mg
Note: High in omega-3 fatty acids.

Tuna (Canned in Water):
Serving Size: 3 ounces (85g)
Calories: 73
Protein: 16g
Cholesterol: 26mg
Note: A convenient source of protein.

Shrimp (Boiled):
Serving Size: 3 ounces (85g)
Calories: 84
Protein: 18g
Cholesterol: 143mg
Note: Low in calories, high in protein.

Trout (Rainbow, Cooked):
Serving Size: 3 ounces (85g)
Calories: 144
Protein: 19g
Cholesterol: 63mg
Note: Contains omega-3 fatty acids.

Cod (Cooked):
Serving Size: 3 ounces (85g)
Calories: 70
Protein: 16g

Cholesterol: 49mg
Note: Low in fat, a lean protein source.

Sardines (Canned in Oil):
Serving Size: 1 can (92g)
Calories: 189
Protein: 22g
Cholesterol: 82mg
Note: Rich in omega-3s and calcium.

Halibut (Cooked):
Serving Size: 3 ounces (85g)
Calories: 77
Protein: 17g
Cholesterol: 35mg
Note: A lean white fish.

Mackerel (Atlantic, Cooked):
Serving Size: 3 ounces (85g)
Calories: 186
Protein: 21g
Cholesterol: 75mg
Note: High in omega-3 fatty acids.

Crab (Cooked):
Serving Size: 3 ounces (85g)
Calories: 97
Protein: 20g
Cholesterol: 95mg
Note: A low-fat protein source.

Lobster (Boiled):
Serving Size: 3 ounces (85g)

Calories: 72
Protein: 16g
Cholesterol: 72mg
Note: Low in calories, a good source of protein.

Catfish (Cooked):
Serving Size: 3 ounces (85g)
Calories: 105
Protein: 20g
Cholesterol: 73mg
Note: A mild-flavored fish.

Clams (Steamed):
Serving Size: 3 ounces (85g)
Calories: 126
Protein: 22g
Cholesterol: 48mg
Note: Rich in iron.

Oysters (Cooked):
Serving Size: 3 ounces (85g)
Calories: 116
Protein: 14g
Cholesterol: 94mg
Note: Good source of zinc.

Scallops (Boiled):
Serving Size: 3 ounces (85g)
Calories: 75
Protein: 15g
Cholesterol: 35mg
Note: Low in fat, high in protein.

Tilapia (Cooked):
Serving Size: 3 ounces (85g)
Calories: 111
Protein: 23g
Cholesterol: 56mg
Note: A mild-flavored white fish.

Meat and poultry

Chicken Breast (Skinless, Cooked):
Serving Size: 3 ounces (85g)
Calories: 142
Protein: 26g
Cholesterol: 73mg
Note: A lean source of protein.

Turkey (Ground, Cooked):
Serving Size: 3 ounces (85g)
Calories: 193
Protein: 22g
Cholesterol: 81mg
Note: Lean ground turkey is a versatile option.

Beef Sirloin (Grilled):
Serving Size: 3 ounces (85g)
Calories: 180
Protein: 25g
Cholesterol: 74mg
Note: A lean cut of beef.

Pork Tenderloin (Roasted):
Serving Size: 3 ounces (85g)
Calories: 122

Protein: 23g
Cholesterol: 64mg
Note: A lean cut of pork.

Lamb Chop (Grilled):
Serving Size: 3 ounces (85g)
Calories: 219
Protein: 23g
Cholesterol: 70mg
Note: Lamb is higher in fat; consumed in moderation.

Ground Beef (90% Lean, Cooked):
Serving Size: 3 ounces (85g)
Calories: 184
Protein: 21g
Cholesterol: 70mg
Note: Choose lean cuts to reduce fat content.

Chicken Thigh (Skinless, Cooked):
Serving Size: 3 ounces (85g)
Calories: 170
Protein: 19g
Cholesterol: 86mg
Note: Dark meat has slightly higher fat content.

Veal Cutlet (Pan-Fried):
Serving Size: 3 ounces (85g)
Calories: 168
Protein: 24g
Cholesterol: 121mg
Note: Veal is higher in cholesterol; consumed in moderation.

Ground Turkey (93% Lean, Cooked):
Serving Size: 3 ounces (85g)
Calories: 176
Protein: 22g
Cholesterol: 76mg
Note: A leaner option than ground beef.

Duck Breast (Roasted):
Serving Size: 3 ounces (85g)
Calories: 165
Protein: 18g
Cholesterol: 82mg
Note: Duck is higher in fat; consumed in moderation.

Chicken Drumstick (Skinless, Cooked):
Serving Size: 3 ounces (85g)
Calories: 174
Protein: 19g
Cholesterol: 92mg
Note: Dark meat is slightly higher in fat.

Ground Lamb (Cooked):
Serving Size: 3 ounces (85g)
Calories: 248
Protein: 17g
Cholesterol: 78mg
Note: Lamb is higher in fat; consumed in moderation.

Turkey Breast (Roasted):
Serving Size: 3 ounces (85g)
Calories: 135
Protein: 30g

Cholesterol: 75mg
Note: A lean source of poultry.

Pork Loin (Roasted):
Serving Size: 3 ounces (85g)
Calories: 122
Protein: 22g
Cholesterol: 64mg
Note: A lean cut of pork.

Chicken Wings (Grilled, Skinless):
Serving Size: 3 ounces (85g)
Calories: 140
Protein: 23g
Cholesterol: 88mg
Note: Choose skinless wings for a lower-fat option.

Low-sodium yogurt

Chobani Non-Fat Greek Yogurt (Plain):
Serving Size: 1 cup (227g)
Calories: 120
Sodium: 65mg
Cholesterol: 10mg
Protein: 22g

Fage Total 0% Greek Yogurt (Plain):
Serving Size: 1 cup (227g)
Calories: 120
Sodium: 80mg
Cholesterol: 10mg
Protein: 23g

Siggi's Icelandic Style Skyr Yogurt (Plain):
Serving Size: 1 cup (240g)
Calories: 100
Sodium: 55mg
Cholesterol: 5mg
Protein: 22g

Stonyfield Organic Low-Fat Yogurt (Plain):
Serving Size: 1 cup (227g)
Calories: 130
Sodium: 80mg
Cholesterol: 15mg
Protein: 12g

Chobani Less Sugar Greek Yogurt (Vanilla):
Serving Size: 1 cup (150g)
Calories: 130
Sodium: 55mg
Cholesterol: 10mg
Protein: 12g

Dannon Oikos Triple Zero Greek Yogurt (Mixed Berry):
Serving Size: 1 container (150g)
Calories: 120
Sodium: 65mg
Cholesterol: 10mg
Protein: 15g

Yoplait Original Yogurt (Strawberry):
Serving Size: 6 ounces (170g)
Calories: 150
Sodium: 70mg
Cholesterol: 15mg
Protein: 5g

Trader Joe's Non-Fat Greek Yogurt (Plain):
Serving Size: 1 cup (227g)
Calories: 120
Sodium: 60mg
Cholesterol: 10mg
Protein: 22g

Oikos Organic Triple Zero Greek Yogurt (Plain):
Serving Size: 1 container (150g)
Calories: 80
Sodium: 55mg

Cholesterol: 0mg
Protein: 15g

Stonyfield Organic Whole Milk Yogurt (Plain):
Serving Size: 1 cup (227g)
Calories: 140
Sodium: 70mg
Cholesterol: 30mg
Protein: 8g

Noosa Yoghurt (Honey):
Serving Size: 8 ounces (227g)
Calories: 280
Sodium: 70mg
Cholesterol: 45mg
Protein: 11g

Dannon Light & Fit Greek Yogurt (Vanilla):
Serving Size: 1 container (150g)
Calories: 80
Sodium: 45mg
Cholesterol: 10mg
Protein: 12g

Chobani Non-Fat Blended Greek Yogurt (Blueberry):
Serving Size: 1 cup (227g)
Calories: 120
Sodium: 85mg
Cholesterol: 5mg
Protein: 15g

So Delicious Dairy Free Coconut Milk Yogurt (Plain):
Serving Size: 1 container (150g)
Calories: 70
Sodium: 15mg
Cholesterol: 0mg
Protein: 1g

Wallaby Organic Greek Low-Fat Yogurt (Strawberry):
Serving Size: 1 container (150g)
Calories: 110
Sodium: 30mg
Cholesterol: 10mg
Protein: 14g

Nuts and seeds

Almonds (Raw):
Serving Size: 1 ounce (28g)
Calories: 160
Sodium: 0mg
Cholesterol: 0mg
Protein: 6g

Walnuts (Raw):
Serving Size: 1 ounce (28g)
Calories: 185
Sodium: 1mg
Cholesterol: 0mg
Protein: 4g

Pistachios (Raw, Unsalted):

Serving Size: 1 ounce (28g)
Calories: 160
Sodium: 0mg
Cholesterol: 0mg
Protein: 6g

Sunflower Seeds (Raw):
Serving Size: 1 ounce (28g)
Calories: 160
Sodium: 1mg
Cholesterol: 0mg
Protein: 6g

Pumpkin Seeds (Raw):
Serving Size: 1 ounce (28g)
Calories: 151
Sodium: 2mg
Cholesterol: 0mg
Protein: 7g

Chia Seeds:
Serving Size: 1 ounce (28g)
Calories: 138
Sodium: 5mg
Cholesterol: 0mg
Protein: 5g

Flaxseeds (Ground):
Serving Size: 1 ounce (28g)
Calories: 151
Sodium: 6mg
Cholesterol: 0mg
Protein: 5g

Cashews (Raw):
Serving Size: 1 ounce (28g)
Calories: 157
Sodium: 3mg
Cholesterol: 0mg
Protein: 5g

Hazelnuts (Raw):
Serving Size: 1 ounce (28g)
Calories: 176
Sodium: 0mg
Cholesterol: 0mg
Protein: 6g

Brazil Nuts (Raw):
Serving Size: 1 ounce (28g)
Calories: 186
Sodium: 1mg
Cholesterol: 0mg
Protein: 4g

Macadamia Nuts (Raw):
Serving Size: 1 ounce (28g)
Calories: 204
Sodium: 1mg
Cholesterol: 0mg
Protein: 2g

Peanuts (Dry Roasted, Unsalted):
Serving Size: 1 ounce (28g)
Calories: 166
Sodium: 2mg
Cholesterol: 0mg

Protein: 7g

Almond Butter (No added salt):
Serving Size: 2 tablespoons (32g)
Calories: 180
Sodium: 0mg
Cholesterol: 0mg
Protein: 6g

Sunflower Butter (No added salt):
Serving Size: 2 tablespoons (32g)
Calories: 200
Sodium: 0mg
Cholesterol: 0mg
Protein: 5g

Hemp Seeds:
Serving Size: 3 tablespoons (30g)
Calories: 170
Sodium: 0mg
Cholesterol: 0mg
Protein: 10g

Eggs

Whole Eggs (Boiled):
Serving Size: 1 large egg (50g)
Calories: 68
Sodium: 62mg
Cholesterol: 186mg
Protein: 6g

Egg Whites (Raw):
Serving Size: 1 large egg white (33g)
Calories: 16
Sodium: 55mg
Cholesterol: 0mg
Protein: 3.6g

Scrambled Eggs (No added salt):
Serving Size: 2 large eggs (124g)
Calories: 174
Sodium: 124mg
Cholesterol: 372mg
Protein: 12g

Hard-Boiled Eggs:
Serving Size: 1 large egg (50g)
Calories: 68
Sodium: 62mg
Cholesterol: 186mg
Protein: 6g

Poached Eggs:
Serving Size: 1 large egg (50g)
Calories: 68
Sodium: 62mg

Cholesterol: 186mg
Protein: 6g

Omelette (No added salt):
Serving Size: 2 large eggs (124g)
Calories: 174
Sodium: 124mg
Cholesterol: 372mg
Protein: 12g

Deviled Eggs (No added salt):
Serving Size: 2 halves (52g)
Calories: 94
Sodium: 112mg
Cholesterol: 371mg
Protein: 6g

Egg Salad (No added salt):
Serving Size: 1 cup (240g)
Calories: 343
Sodium: 290mg
Cholesterol: 778mg
Protein: 26g

Frittata (No added salt):
Serving Size: 1 slice (100g)
Calories: 142
Sodium: 108mg
Cholesterol: 372mg
Protein: 12g

Soft-Boiled Eggs:
Serving Size: 1 large egg (50g)

Calories: 68
Sodium: 62mg
Cholesterol: 186mg
Protein: 6g

Egg Muffins (No added salt):
Serving Size: 2 muffins (124g)
Calories: 174
Sodium: 124mg
Cholesterol: 372mg
Protein: 12g

Egg Drop Soup (No added salt):
Serving Size: 1 cup (240g)
Calories: 68
Sodium: 53mg
Cholesterol: 164mg
Protein: 7g

Baked Eggs (No added salt):
Serving Size: 2 large eggs (124g)
Calories: 174
Sodium: 124mg
Cholesterol: 372mg
Protein: 12g

Egg Casserole (No added salt):
Serving Size: 1 cup (240g)
Calories: 270
Sodium: 176mg
Cholesterol: 419mg
Protein: 20g

Egg and Vegetable Stir-Fry (No added salt):
Serving Size: 1 cup (240g)
Calories: 184
Sodium: 121mg
Cholesterol: 372mg
Protein: 15g

Lean meats and poultry

Chicken Breast (Skinless, Grilled):
Serving Size: 3 ounces (85g)
Calories: 165
Sodium: 74mg
Cholesterol: 74mg
Protein: 31g

Turkey Breast (Roasted):
Serving Size: 3 ounces (85g)
Calories: 135
Sodium: 50mg
Cholesterol: 50mg
Protein: 30g

Pork Tenderloin (Roasted):
Serving Size: 3 ounces (85g)
Calories: 122
Sodium: 49mg
Cholesterol: 62mg
Protein: 22g

Beef Sirloin (Grilled):
Serving Size: 3 ounces (85g)
Calories: 180

Sodium: 45mg
Cholesterol: 64mg
Protein: 25g

Ground Turkey (93% Lean, Cooked):
Serving Size: 3 ounces (85g)
Calories: 176
Sodium: 70mg
Cholesterol: 76mg
Protein: 22g

Chicken Thigh (Skinless, Roasted):
Serving Size: 3 ounces (85g)
Calories: 180
Sodium: 70mg
Cholesterol: 100mg
Protein: 21g

Veal Cutlet (Pan-Fried):
Serving Size: 3 ounces (85g)
Calories: 168
Sodium: 68mg
Cholesterol: 120mg
Protein: 24g

Ground Chicken (Cooked):
Serving Size: 3 ounces (85g)
Calories: 165
Sodium: 80mg
Cholesterol: 75mg
Protein: 21g

Ground Beef (90% Lean, Cooked):
Serving Size: 3 ounces (85g)
Calories: 184
Sodium: 70mg
Cholesterol: 70mg
Protein: 21g

Lamb Chop (Grilled):
Serving Size: 3 ounces (85g)
Calories: 219
Sodium: 60mg
Cholesterol: 70mg
Protein: 23g

Chicken Drumstick (Skinless, Roasted):
Serving Size: 3 ounces (85g)
Calories: 174
Sodium: 76mg
Cholesterol: 105mg
Protein: 19g

Ground Veal (Cooked):
Serving Size: 3 ounces (85g)
Calories: 191
Sodium: 77mg
Cholesterol: 136mg
Protein: 21g

Chicken Wing (Grilled, Skinless):
Serving Size: 3 ounces (85g)
Calories: 140
Sodium: 62mg
Cholesterol: 88mg

Protein: 23g

Ground Pork (Cooked):
Serving Size: 3 ounces (85g)
Calories: 231
Sodium: 55mg
Cholesterol: 79mg
Protein: 22g

Turkey Burger (No added salt, Grilled):
Serving Size: 1 patty (112g)
Calories: 170
Sodium: 75mg
Cholesterol: 85mg
Protein: 20g

Beans and lentils

Black Beans (Canned, No Salt Added):
Serving Size: 1/2 cup (130g)
Calories: 110
Sodium: 15mg
Cholesterol: 0mg
Protein: 7g

Kidney Beans (Canned, No Salt Added):
Serving Size: 1/2 cup (130g)
Calories: 110
Sodium: 15mg
Cholesterol: 0mg
Protein: 7g

Chickpeas (Canned, No Salt Added):
Serving Size: 1/2 cup (130g)
Calories: 120
Sodium: 5mg
Cholesterol: 0mg
Protein: 6g

Lentils (Cooked, No Salt Added):
Serving Size: 1/2 cup (99g)
Calories: 115
Sodium: 2mg
Cholesterol: 0mg
Protein: 9g

Pinto Beans (Canned, No Salt Added):
Serving Size: 1/2 cup (130g)
Calories: 120
Sodium: 5mg
Cholesterol: 0mg
Protein: 7g

Cannellini Beans (Canned, No Salt Added):
Serving Size: 1/2 cup (130g)
Calories: 100
Sodium: 5mg
Cholesterol: 0mg
Protein: 7g

Black-eyed Peas (Canned, No Salt Added):
Serving Size: 1/2 cup (130g)
Calories: 70
Sodium: 5mg
Cholesterol: 0mg

Protein: 4g

Garbanzo Beans (Canned, No Salt Added):
Serving Size: 1/2 cup (130g)
Calories: 120
Sodium: 5mg
Cholesterol: 0mg
Protein: 6g

Split Peas (Cooked, No Salt Added):
Serving Size: 1/2 cup (98g)
Calories: 70
Sodium: 0mg
Cholesterol: 0mg
Protein: 5g

Adzuki Beans (Canned, No Salt Added):
Serving Size: 1/2 cup (130g)
Calories: 100
Sodium: 0mg
Cholesterol: 0mg
Protein: 6g

Great Northern Beans (Canned, No Salt Added):
Serving Size: 1/2 cup (130g)
Calories: 90
Sodium: 5mg
Cholesterol: 0mg
Protein: 6g

Lima Beans (Frozen, No Salt Added):
Serving Size: 1/2 cup (95g)
Calories: 60

Sodium: 0mg
Cholesterol: 0mg
Protein: 4g

Black Lentils (Cooked, No Salt Added):
Serving Size: 1/2 cup (100g)
Calories: 110
Sodium: 0mg
Cholesterol: 0mg
Protein: 9g

Mung Beans (Cooked, No Salt Added):
Serving Size: 1/2 cup (104g)
Calories: 100
Sodium: 0mg
Cholesterol: 0mg
Protein: 7g

Red Kidney Beans (Canned, No Salt Added):
Serving Size: 1/2 cup (130g)
Calories: 110
Sodium: 5mg
Cholesterol: 0mg
Protein: 7g

Quinoa (Cooked, No Salt Added):
Serving Size: 1 cup (185g)
Calories: 222
Sodium: 13mg
Cholesterol: 0mg
Protein: 8g

Brown Rice (Cooked, No Salt Added):
Serving Size: 1 cup (195g)
Calories: 215
Sodium: 5mg
Cholesterol: 0mg
Protein: 5g

Bulgur (Cooked, No Salt Added):
Serving Size: 1 cup (182g)
Calories: 151
Sodium: 7mg
Cholesterol: 0mg
Protein: 5g

Barley (Cooked, No Salt Added):
Serving Size: 1 cup (157g)
Calories: 193
Sodium: 5mg
Cholesterol: 0mg
Protein: 4g

Millet (Cooked, No Salt Added):
Serving Size: 1 cup (174g)
Calories: 207
Sodium: 2mg

Cholesterol: 0mg
Protein: 6g

Oats (Cooked, No Salt Added):
Serving Size: 1 cup (234g)
Calories: 145
Sodium: 2mg
Cholesterol: 0mg
Protein: 6g

Farro (Cooked, No Salt Added):
Serving Size: 1 cup (194g)
Calories: 220
Sodium: 5mg
Cholesterol: 0mg
Protein: 7g

Whole Wheat Pasta (Cooked, No Salt Added):
Serving Size: 1 cup (140g)
Calories: 174
Sodium: 3mg
Cholesterol: 0mg
Protein: 7g

Freekeh (Cooked, No Salt Added):
Serving Size: 1 cup (174g)
Calories: 290
Sodium: 7mg
Cholesterol: 0mg
Protein: 12g

Wild Rice (Cooked, No Salt Added):
Serving Size: 1 cup (164g)
Calories: 166
Sodium: 7mg
Cholesterol: 0mg
Protein: 6g

Sorghum (Cooked, No Salt Added):
Serving Size: 1 cup (192g)
Calories: 220
Sodium: 2mg
Cholesterol: 0mg
Protein: 10g

Whole Wheat Bread (1 slice):
Serving Size: 1 slice (28g)
Calories: 69
Sodium: 77mg
Cholesterol: 0mg
Protein: 3g

Amaranth (Cooked, No Salt Added):
Serving Size: 1 cup (246g)
Calories: 251
Sodium: 7mg
Cholesterol: 0mg
Protein: 9g

Brown Rice Cakes (1 cake):
Serving Size: 1 cake (9g)
Calories: 35
Sodium: 0mg
Cholesterol: 0mg

Protein: 1g

Buckwheat (Cooked, No Salt Added):
Serving Size: 1 cup (168g)
Calories: 155
Sodium: 5mg
Cholesterol: 0mg
Protein: 6g

Fruits

Apple (Medium):
Serving Size: 1 medium apple (182g)
Calories: 95
Sodium: 0mg
Cholesterol: 0mg
Dietary Fiber: 4g

Banana (Medium):
Serving Size: 1 medium banana (118g)
Calories: 105
Sodium: 1mg
Cholesterol: 0mg
Dietary Fiber: 3g

Orange (Medium):
Serving Size: 1 medium orange (131g)
Calories: 62
Sodium: 0mg
Cholesterol: 0mg
Dietary Fiber: 3g

Strawberries (1 cup, sliced):
Serving Size: 1 cup (166g)
Calories: 50
Sodium: 2mg
Cholesterol: 0mg
Dietary Fiber: 8g

Watermelon (1 cup, diced):
Serving Size: 1 cup (152g)
Calories: 46
Sodium: 2mg
Cholesterol: 0mg
Dietary Fiber: 1g

Grapes (1 cup, seedless):
Serving Size: 1 cup (151g)
Calories: 104
Sodium: 2mg
Cholesterol: 0mg
Dietary Fiber: 1g

Pineapple (1 cup, chunks):
Serving Size: 1 cup (165g)
Calories: 83
Sodium: 2mg
Cholesterol: 0mg
Dietary Fiber: 2g

Kiwi (Medium):
Serving Size: 1 medium kiwi (100g)
Calories: 61
Sodium: 3mg
Cholesterol: 0mg

Dietary Fiber: 2g

Peach (Medium):
Serving Size: 1 medium peach (150g)
Calories: 60
Sodium: 0mg
Cholesterol: 0mg
Dietary Fiber: 2g

Cantaloupe (1 cup, cubes):
Serving Size: 1 cup (177g)
Calories: 54
Sodium: 14mg
Cholesterol: 0mg
Dietary Fiber: 2g

Blueberries (1 cup):
Serving Size: 1 cup (148g)
Calories: 84
Sodium: 1mg
Cholesterol: 0mg
Dietary Fiber: 3g

Mango (1 cup, diced):
Serving Size: 1 cup (165g)
Calories: 99
Sodium: 1mg
Cholesterol: 0mg
Dietary Fiber: 3g

Raspberry (1 cup):
Serving Size: 1 cup (123g)
Calories: 64

Sodium: 1mg
Cholesterol: 0mg
Dietary Fiber: 8g

Pear (Medium):
Serving Size: 1 medium pear (178g)
Calories: 101
Sodium: 1mg
Cholesterol: 0mg
Dietary Fiber: 6g

Plum (2 medium):
Serving Size: 2 medium plums (151g)
Calories: 60
Sodium: 0mg
Cholesterol: 0mg
Dietary Fiber: 2g

Vegetables

Broccoli (1 cup, cooked):
Serving Size: 1 cup (156g)
Calories: 55
Sodium: 60mg
Cholesterol: 0mg
Dietary Fiber: 5g

Spinach (1 cup, cooked):
Serving Size: 1 cup (180g)
Calories: 41
Sodium: 24mg
Cholesterol: 0mg
Dietary Fiber: 6g

Carrots (1 cup, cooked):
Serving Size: 1 cup (156g)
Calories: 54
Sodium: 88mg
Cholesterol: 0mg
Dietary Fiber: 5g

Cauliflower (1 cup, cooked):
Serving Size: 1 cup (155g)
Calories: 29
Sodium: 30mg
Cholesterol: 0mg
Dietary Fiber: 3g

Bell Peppers (1 cup, raw):
Serving Size: 1 cup (149g)
Calories: 46
Sodium: 3mg
Cholesterol: 0mg
Dietary Fiber: 3g

Zucchini (1 cup, cooked):
Serving Size: 1 cup (196g)
Calories: 21
Sodium: 9mg
Cholesterol: 0mg
Dietary Fiber: 2g

Cabbage (1 cup, cooked):
Serving Size: 1 cup (150g)
Calories: 44
Sodium: 20mg

Cholesterol: 0mg
Dietary Fiber: 3g

Kale (1 cup, cooked):
Serving Size: 1 cup (130g)
Calories: 36
Sodium: 23mg
Cholesterol: 0mg
Dietary Fiber: 5g

Asparagus (1 cup, cooked):
Serving Size: 1 cup (180g)
Calories: 43
Sodium: 2mg
Cholesterol: 0mg
Dietary Fiber: 5g

Brussels Sprouts (1 cup, cooked):
Serving Size: 1 cup (156g)
Calories: 56
Sodium: 23mg
Cholesterol: 0mg
Dietary Fiber: 6g

Cucumber (1 cup, sliced):
Serving Size: 1 cup (104g)
Calories: 16
Sodium: 2mg
Cholesterol: 0mg
Dietary Fiber: 1g

Green Beans (1 cup, cooked):
Serving Size: 1 cup (125g)

Calories: 44
Sodium: 5mg
Cholesterol: 0mg
Dietary Fiber: 4g

Sweet Potatoes (1 medium, baked):
Serving Size: 1 medium sweet potato (114g)
Calories: 103
Sodium: 68mg
Cholesterol: 0mg
Dietary Fiber: 4g

Onions (1 cup, raw):
Serving Size: 1 cup (160g)
Calories: 64
Sodium: 5mg
Cholesterol: 0mg
Dietary Fiber: 3g

Tomatoes (1 medium):
Serving Size: 1 medium tomato (182g)
Calories: 22
Sodium: 6mg
Cholesterol: 0mg
Dietary Fiber: 2g

Unsweetened herbal tea

Peppermint Tea (1 tea bag):
Serving Size: 1 tea bag (2g)
Calories: 0
Sodium: 0mg
Cholesterol: 0mg

Chamomile Tea (1 tea bag):
Serving Size: 1 tea bag (2g)
Calories: 0
Sodium: 0mg
Cholesterol: 0mg

Hibiscus Tea (1 tea bag):
Serving Size: 1 tea bag (2g)
Calories: 0
Sodium: 0mg
Cholesterol: 0mg

Ginger Tea (1 tea bag):
Serving Size: 1 tea bag (2g)
Calories: 0
Sodium: 0mg
Cholesterol: 0mg

Lemon Balm Tea (1 tea bag):
Serving Size: 1 tea bag (2g)
Calories: 0
Sodium: 0mg
Cholesterol: 0mg

Dandelion Tea (1 tea bag):
Serving Size: 1 tea bag (2g)

Calories: 0
Sodium: 0mg
Cholesterol: 0mg

Rosehip Tea (1 tea bag):
Serving Size: 1 tea bag (2g)
Calories: 0
Sodium: 0mg
Cholesterol: 0mg

Nettle Tea (1 tea bag):
Serving Size: 1 tea bag (2g)
Calories: 0
Sodium: 0mg
Cholesterol: 0mg

Lavender Tea (1 tea bag):
Serving Size: 1 tea bag (2g)
Calories: 0
Sodium: 0mg
Cholesterol: 0mg

Cinnamon Tea (1 tea bag):
Serving Size: 1 tea bag (2g)
Calories: 0
Sodium: 0mg
Cholesterol: 0mg

Chai Tea (1 tea bag):
Serving Size: 1 tea bag (2g)
Calories: 0
Sodium: 0mg
Cholesterol: 0mg

Fennel Tea (1 tea bag):
Serving Size: 1 tea bag (2g)
Calories: 0
Sodium: 0mg
Cholesterol: 0mg

Echinacea Tea (1 tea bag):
Serving Size: 1 tea bag (2g)
Calories: 0
Sodium: 0mg
Cholesterol: 0mg

Lemongrass Tea (1 tea bag):
Serving Size: 1 tea bag (2g)
Calories: 0
Sodium: 0mg
Cholesterol: 0mg

Turmeric Tea (1 tea bag):
Serving Size: 1 tea bag (2g)
Calories: 0
Sodium: 0mg
Cholesterol: 0mg

Stevia (1 packet):
Serving Size: 1 packet (1g)
Calories: 0
Sodium: 0mg
Cholesterol: 0mg

Monk Fruit Sweetener (1 teaspoon):
Serving Size: 1 teaspoon (0.5g)
Calories: 0
Sodium: 0mg
Cholesterol: 0mg

Erythritol (1 teaspoon):
Serving Size: 1 teaspoon (4g)
Calories: 0
Sodium: 0mg
Cholesterol: 0mg

Xylitol (1 teaspoon):
Serving Size: 1 teaspoon (4g)
Calories: 10
Sodium: 0mg
Cholesterol: 0mg

Agave Nectar (1 tablespoon):
Serving Size: 1 tablespoon (21g)
Calories: 60
Sodium: 0mg
Cholesterol: 0mg

Sucralose (1 packet):
Serving Size: 1 packet (1g)

Calories: 0
Sodium: 0mg
Cholesterol: 0mg

Aspartame (1 packet):
Serving Size: 1 packet (1g)
Calories: 0
Sodium: 0mg
Cholesterol: 0mg

Saccharin (1 packet):
Serving Size: 1 packet (1g)
Calories: 0
Sodium: 0mg
Cholesterol: 0mg

Maple Syrup, Pure (1 tablespoon):
Serving Size: 1 tablespoon (20g)
Calories: 52
Sodium: 1mg
Cholesterol: 0mg

Honey (1 tablespoon):
Serving Size: 1 tablespoon (21g)
Calories: 64
Sodium: 1mg
Cholesterol: 0mg

Coconut Sugar (1 teaspoon):
Serving Size: 1 teaspoon (4g)
Calories: 15
Sodium: 0mg
Cholesterol: 0mg

Date Syrup (1 tablespoon):
Serving Size: 1 tablespoon (20g)
Calories: 60
Sodium: 0mg
Cholesterol: 0mg

Brown Rice Syrup (1 tablespoon):
Serving Size: 1 tablespoon (20g)
Calories: 55
Sodium: 0mg
Cholesterol: 0mg

Sorbitol (1 teaspoon):
Serving Size: 1 teaspoon (4g)
Calories: 10
Sodium: 0mg
Cholesterol: 0mg

Molasses (1 tablespoon):
Serving Size: 1 tablespoon (20g)
Calories: 58
Sodium: 10mg
Cholesterol: 0mg

Beverages

Water (1 cup):
Serving Size: 1 cup (240ml)
Calories: 0
Sodium: 0mg
Cholesterol: 0mg

Herbal Tea (unsweetened, 1 cup):
Serving Size: 1 cup (240ml)
Calories: 0
Sodium: 0mg
Cholesterol: 0mg

Black Coffee (unsweetened, 1 cup):
Serving Size: 1 cup (240ml)
Calories: 2
Sodium: 5mg
Cholesterol: 0mg

Green Tea (unsweetened, 1 cup):
Serving Size: 1 cup (240ml)
Calories: 0
Sodium: 0mg
Cholesterol: 0mg

Almond Milk (unsweetened, 1 cup):
Serving Size: 1 cup (240ml)
Calories: 30
Sodium: 180mg
Cholesterol: 0mg

Coconut Water (unsweetened, 1 cup):
Serving Size: 1 cup (240ml)

Calories: 46
Sodium: 252mg
Cholesterol: 0mg

Tomato Juice (low-sodium, 1 cup):
Serving Size: 1 cup (240ml)
Calories: 41
Sodium: 24mg
Cholesterol: 0mg

Vegetable Juice (low-sodium, 1 cup):
Serving Size: 1 cup (240ml)
Calories: 50
Sodium: 140mg
Cholesterol: 0mg

Sparkling Water (unsweetened, 1 cup):
Serving Size: 1 cup (240ml)
Calories: 0
Sodium: 0mg
Cholesterol: 0mg

Lemonade (homemade, unsweetened, 1 cup):
Serving Size: 1 cup (240ml)
Calories: 4
Sodium: 3mg
Cholesterol: 0mg

Orange Juice (fresh, unsweetened, 1 cup):
Serving Size: 1 cup (240ml)
Calories: 112
Sodium: 2mg
Cholesterol: 0mg

Pomegranate Juice (unsweetened, 1 cup):
Serving Size: 1 cup (240ml)
Calories: 134
Sodium: 10mg
Cholesterol: 0mg

Rooibos Tea (unsweetened, 1 cup):
Serving Size: 1 cup (240ml)
Calories: 0
Sodium: 0mg
Cholesterol: 0mg

Ginger Tea (unsweetened, 1 cup):
Serving Size: 1 cup (240ml)
Calories: 0
Sodium: 1mg
Cholesterol: 0mg

Mint Tea (unsweetened, 1 cup):
Serving Size: 1 cup (240ml)
Calories: 0
Sodium: 1mg
Cholesterol: 0mg

Baking Powder (1 teaspoon):
Serving Size: 1 teaspoon (4g)
Calories: 0
Sodium: 500mg
Cholesterol: 0mg

Baking Soda (1 teaspoon):
Serving Size: 1 teaspoon (4g)
Calories: 0
Sodium: 0mg
Cholesterol: 0mg

Cream of Tartar (1 teaspoon):
Serving Size: 1 teaspoon (3g)
Calories: 0
Sodium: 1mg
Cholesterol: 0mg

Unsalted Butter (1 tablespoon):
Serving Size: 1 tablespoon (14g)
Calories: 102
Sodium: 2mg
Cholesterol: 31mg

Olive Oil (1 tablespoon):
Serving Size: 1 tablespoon (14g)
Calories: 120
Sodium: 0mg
Cholesterol: 0mg

Coconut Oil (1 tablespoon):
Serving Size: 1 tablespoon (13.6g)

Calories: 121
Sodium: 0mg
Cholesterol: 0mg

Honey (1 tablespoon):
Serving Size: 1 tablespoon (21g)
Calories: 64
Sodium: 1mg
Cholesterol: 0mg

Maple Syrup, Pure (1 tablespoon):
Serving Size: 1 tablespoon (20g)
Calories: 52
Sodium: 1mg
Cholesterol: 0mg

Vanilla Extract (1 teaspoon):
Serving Size: 1 teaspoon (4g)
Calories: 12
Sodium: 0mg
Cholesterol: 0mg

Almond Extract (1 teaspoon):
Serving Size: 1 teaspoon (4g)
Calories: 12
Sodium: 0mg
Cholesterol: 0mg

Unsalted Chicken or Vegetable Broth (1 cup):
Serving Size: 1 cup (240ml)
Calories: 5
Sodium: 5mg
Cholesterol: 0mg

Garlic Powder (1 teaspoon):
Serving Size: 1 teaspoon (3g)
Calories: 10
Sodium: 0mg
Cholesterol: 0mg

Onion Powder (1 teaspoon):
Serving Size: 1 teaspoon (3g)
Calories: 10
Sodium: 0mg
Cholesterol: 0mg

Black Pepper (1 teaspoon):
Serving Size: 1 teaspoon (2g)
Calories: 6
Sodium: 0mg
Cholesterol: 0mg

Unsalted Tomato Paste (2 tablespoons):
Serving Size: 2 tablespoons (33g)
Calories: 30
Sodium: 20mg
Cholesterol: 0mg

Protein Sources

Chicken Breast (cooked, skinless, 3 ounces):
Serving Size: 3 ounces (85g)
Calories: 142
Sodium: 74mg
Cholesterol: 73mg
Protein: 26g

Turkey Breast (cooked, skinless, 3 ounces):
Serving Size: 3 ounces (85g)
Calories: 135
Sodium: 50mg
Cholesterol: 49mg
Protein: 30g

Salmon (cooked, 3 ounces):
Serving Size: 3 ounces (85g)
Calories: 206
Sodium: 50mg
Cholesterol: 67mg
Protein: 22g

Tofu (firm, 3 ounces):
Serving Size: 3 ounces (85g)
Calories: 70
Sodium: 8mg
Cholesterol: 0mg
Protein: 8g

Eggs (boiled, 1 large):
Serving Size: 1 large egg (50g)
Calories: 68
Sodium: 68mg

Cholesterol: 186mg
Protein: 6g

Lentils (cooked, 1 cup):
Serving Size: 1 cup (198g)
Calories: 230
Sodium: 5mg
Cholesterol: 0mg
Protein: 18g

Chickpeas (canned, drained, 1 cup):
Serving Size: 1 cup (240g)
Calories: 269
Sodium: 11mg
Cholesterol: 0mg
Protein: 15g

Greek Yogurt (plain, non-fat, 1 cup):
Serving Size: 1 cup (240g)
Calories: 100
Sodium: 73mg
Cholesterol: 5mg
Protein: 22g

Cottage Cheese (low-fat, 1 cup):
Serving Size: 1 cup (240g)
Calories: 206
Sodium: 918mg
Cholesterol: 15mg
Protein: 28g

Quinoa (cooked, 1 cup):
Serving Size: 1 cup (185g)
Calories: 222
Sodium: 13mg
Cholesterol: 0mg
Protein: 8g

White Beans (canned, drained, 1 cup):
Serving Size: 1 cup (240g)
Calories: 248
Sodium: 1mg
Cholesterol: 0mg
Protein: 19g

Hummus (2 tablespoons):
Serving Size: 2 tablespoons (28g)
Calories: 50
Sodium: 58mg
Cholesterol: 0mg
Protein: 2g

Peanut Butter (2 tablespoons):
Serving Size: 2 tablespoons (32g)
Calories: 190
Sodium: 140mg
Cholesterol: 0mg
Protein: 8g

Ground Turkey (cooked, 3 ounces):
Serving Size: 3 ounces (85g)
Calories: 193
Sodium: 76mg
Cholesterol: 85mg

Protein: 22gSoy Milk (unsweetened, 1 cup):
Serving Size: 1 cup (240ml)
Calories: 80
Sodium: 60mg
Cholesterol: 0mg
Protein: 7g

kidney-friendly renal diet Meal Plan

Breakfast

1. Vegetable Omelette:
Ingredients:
2 large eggs
1/4 cup diced bell peppers
1/4 cup diced tomatoes
1/4 cup chopped spinach
1 tablespoon olive oil

Preparation:
Whisk eggs in a bowl.
Heat olive oil in a non-stick pan.
Add vegetables to the pan and sauté until tender.
Pour whisked eggs over the vegetables and cook until set.
Nutritional Information (Approx):
Calories: 250
Protein: 15g
Sodium: 150mg
Potassium: 400mg

2. Quinoa Breakfast Bowl:
Ingredients:
1/2 cup cooked quinoa
1/4 cup sliced strawberries
1/4 cup blueberries
1 tablespoon chopped almonds
1 tablespoon honey

Preparation:
Cook quinoa according to package instructions.
Combine cooked quinoa with berries and almonds.
Drizzle honey on top.
Nutritional Information (Approx):
Calories: 300
Protein: 8g
Sodium: 5mg
Potassium: 200mg

3. Greek Yogurt Parfait:
Ingredients:
1/2 cup low-fat Greek yogurt
1/4 cup granola (low-sodium)
1/4 cup mixed berries
1 tablespoon chia seeds

Preparation:
Layer Greek yogurt, granola, berries, and chia seeds
in a glass.
Repeat layers.
Nutritional Information (Approx):
Calories: 280
Protein: 15g

Sodium: 80mg
Potassium: 220mg

4. Sweet Potato Hash:
Ingredients:
1 medium sweet potato, grated
1/4 cup diced onions
1/4 cup diced bell peppers
1 tablespoon olive oil

Preparation:
Heat olive oil in a skillet.
Add grated sweet potato, onions, and bell peppers.
Sauté until sweet potatoes are cooked.
Nutritional Information (Approx):
Calories: 220
Protein: 4g
Sodium: 30mg
Potassium: 380mg

5. Smoothie Bowl:
Ingredients:
1/2 cup frozen mixed berries
1/2 banana
1/2 cup low-fat milk or dairy-free alternative
1 tablespoon flax seeds

Preparation:
Blend berries, banana, and milk until smooth.
Pour into a bowl and top with flaxseeds.
Nutritional Information (Approx):
Calories: 200
Protein: 6g

Sodium: 50mg
Potassium: 350mg

Lunch

1. Grilled Salmon with Quinoa and Steamed Vegetables:
Ingredients:
4 oz grilled salmon
1/2 cup cooked quinoa
1 cup steamed broccoli and carrots
1 tablespoon olive oil

Preparation:
Grill salmon until fully cooked.
Cook quinoa according to package instructions.
Steam broccoli and carrots.
Drizzle olive oil over the vegetables.
Nutritional Information (Approx):
Calories: 400
Protein: 30g
Sodium: 80mg
Potassium: 600mg

2. Turkey and Veggie Wrap:
Ingredients:
3 oz low-sodium deli turkey
1 whole wheat tortilla
1/4 cup hummus
1/4 cup shredded lettuce
1/4 cup diced tomatoes

Preparation:
Spread hummus on the whole wheat tortilla.
Layer turkey, lettuce, and tomatoes.
Roll into a wrap.
Nutritional Information (Approx):
Calories: 320
Protein: 25g
Sodium: 350mg
Potassium: 280mg

3. Vegetarian Lentil Soup:
Ingredients:
1 cup cooked lentils
1/2 cup diced carrots
1/2 cup diced celery
1/2 cup diced onions
2 cups low-sodium vegetable broth

Preparation:
Cook lentils according to package instructions.
In a pot, combine lentils, carrots, celery, onions, and
vegetable broth.
Simmer until vegetables are tender.
Nutritional Information (Approx):
Calories: 250
Protein: 18g
Sodium: 150mg
Potassium: 400mg

4. Quinoa Salad with Chicken:
Ingredients:
3 oz grilled chicken breast, sliced
1/2 cup cooked quinoa

1/4 cup cherry tomatoes, halved
1/4 cup cucumber, diced
2 tablespoons balsamic vinaigrette

Preparation:
Grill chicken until fully cooked.
In a bowl, combine quinoa, chicken, tomatoes, cucumber, and vinaigrette.
Nutritional Information (Approx):
Calories: 350
Protein: 30g
Sodium: 120mg
Potassium: 400mg

5. Baked Cod with Sweet Potato Fries:
Ingredients:
4 oz baked cod
1 medium sweet potato, cut into fries
1 tablespoon olive oil
1/4 teaspoon garlic powder

Preparation:
Bake cod in the oven until fully cooked.
Toss sweet potato fries in olive oil and sprinkle with garlic powder.
Bake sweet potato fries until crispy.
Nutritional Information (Approx):
Calories: 380
Protein: 30g
Sodium: 90mg
Potassium: 600mg

Dinner

1. Grilled Chicken Stir-Fry:
Ingredients:
4 oz grilled chicken breast, sliced
1/2 cup broccoli florets
1/2 cup snap peas
1/2 cup bell peppers, sliced
1 tablespoon low-sodium soy sauce

Preparation:
Grill chicken until fully cooked.
In a pan, stir-fry broccoli, snap peas, and bell peppers.
Add sliced chicken and soy sauce.
Nutritional Information (Approx):
Calories: 300
Protein: 30g
Sodium: 300mg
Potassium: 400mg

2. Salmon and Asparagus Bake:
Ingredients:
4 oz baked salmon fillet
1 cup asparagus spears
1 tablespoon olive oil
Lemon slices for garnish

Preparation:
Place salmon on a baking sheet.
Arrange asparagus around the salmon.
Drizzle olive oil over salmon and asparagus.
Bake until salmon is cooked through.
Nutritional Information (Approx):

Calories: 350
Protein: 30g
Sodium: 70mg
Potassium: 600mg

3. Vegetarian Stuffed Bell Peppers:
Ingredients:
2 bell peppers, halved
1/2 cup cooked brown rice
1/2 cup black beans, canned (low-sodium)
1/4 cup corn kernels
1/4 cup salsa

Preparation:
Preheat the oven to 375°F (190°C).
Mix cooked rice, black beans, corn, and salsa in a
bowl.
Stuff bell pepper halves with the mixture.
Bake until peppers are tender.
Nutritional Information (Approx):
Calories: 320
Protein: 12g
Sodium: 180mg
Potassium: 350mg

4. Eggplant and Tomato Bake:
Ingredients:
1 medium-sized eggplant, sliced
1 cup cherry tomatoes, halved
2 tablespoons olive oil
1/2 teaspoon dried oregano

Preparation:
Preheat the oven to 400°F (200°C).
Arrange eggplant slices on a baking sheet.
Place cherry tomatoes on top.
Drizzle with olive oil and sprinkle with oregano.
Bake until the eggplant is tender.
Nutritional Information (Approx):
Calories: 250
Protein: 5g
Sodium: 10mg
Potassium: 400mg

5. Shrimp and Zucchini Noodles:
Ingredients:
4 oz shrimp, peeled and deveined
1 medium zucchini, spiralized
1/4 cup cherry tomatoes, halved
1 tablespoon olive oil
1/2 teaspoon garlic powder

Preparation:
Sauté shrimp in olive oil until cooked.
Add zucchini noodles and cherry tomatoes.
Sprinkle with garlic powder and cook until vegetables are tender.
Nutritional Information (Approx):
Calories: 280
Protein: 25g
Sodium: 150mg
Potassium: 350mg

1. Fruit Salad with Mint:
Ingredients:
1/2 cup melon cubes
1/2 cup berries (strawberries, blueberries, or raspberries)
1/2 cup pineapple chunks
Fresh mint leaves for garnish

Preparation:
Combine melon cubes, berries, and pineapple in a bowl.
Garnish with fresh mint leaves.
Nutritional Information (Approx):
Calories: 50
Protein: 1g
Sodium: 5mg
Potassium: 150mg

2. Greek Yogurt Parfait with Berries:
Ingredients:
1/2 cup low-fat Greek yogurt
1/4 cup granola (low-sodium)
1/4 cup mixed berries
1 tablespoon honey (optional)

Preparation:
In a glass, layer Greek yogurt, granola, and berries.
Drizzle honey on top if desired.
Nutritional Information (Approx):
Calories: 200
Protein: 10g
Sodium: 60mg

Potassium: 200mg

3. Baked Apples with Cinnamon:
Ingredients:
1 apple, cored and sliced
1/2 teaspoon cinnamon
1 tablespoon chopped walnuts (optional)

Preparation:
Preheat the oven to 375°F (190°C).
Place apple slices in a baking dish and sprinkle with
cinnamon.
Bake until apples are tender.
Top with chopped walnuts if desired.
Nutritional Information (Approx):
Calories: 100
Protein: 1g
Sodium: 0mg
Potassium: 100mg

4. Coconut Chia Pudding:
Ingredients:
2 tablespoons chia seeds
1/2 cup unsweetened coconut milk
1/4 teaspoon vanilla extract
1 tablespoon shredded coconut (unsweetened)

Preparation:
In a bowl, mix chia seeds, coconut milk, and vanilla
extract.
Refrigerate for at least 2 hours or overnight.
Top with shredded coconut before serving.
Nutritional Information (Approx):

Calories: 150
Protein: 3g
Sodium: 10mg
Potassium: 50mg

5. Berry Sorbet:
Ingredients:
1 cup mixed berries (strawberries, blueberries, or raspberries)
1 tablespoon lemon juice
1 tablespoon honey (optional)

Preparation:
Blend mixed berries, lemon juice, and honey until smooth.
Pour into a shallow dish and freeze for 4-6 hours, stirring occasionally.
Nutritional Information (Approx):
Calories: 80
Protein: 1g
Sodium: 0mg
Potassium: 150mg

Snacks

1. Cucumber and Hummus Slices:
Ingredients:
1 medium cucumber, sliced
2 tablespoons hummus (low-sodium)

Preparation:
Slice the cucumber into rounds.
Dip cucumber slices into hummus.
Nutritional Information (Approx):

Calories: 50
Protein: 2g
Sodium: 50mg
Potassium: 150mg

2. Rice Cake with Almond Butter:
Ingredients:
1 rice cake (low-sodium)
1 tablespoon almond butter

Preparation:
Spread almond butter on the rice cake.
Nutritional Information (Approx):
Calories: 100
Protein: 3g
Sodium: 0mg
Potassium: 50mg

3. Vegetable Sticks with Greek Yogurt Dip:
Ingredients:
1/2 cup carrot sticks
1/2 cup cucumber sticks
1/2 cup bell pepper strips
1/2 cup cherry tomatoes
1/2 cup low-fat Greek yogurt

Preparation:
Arrange vegetable sticks on a plate.
Use Greek yogurt as a dip.
Nutritional Information (Approx):
Calories: 80
Protein: 4g
Sodium: 30mg

Potassium: 300mg

4. Hard-Boiled Egg and Whole Grain Crackers:
Ingredients:
1 hard-boiled egg
5-6 whole grain crackers

Preparation:
Peel and slice the hard-boiled egg.
Serve with whole grain crackers.
Nutritional Information (Approx):
Calories: 150
Protein: 8g
Sodium: 70mg
Potassium: 70mg

5. Mixed Berries with Cottage Cheese:
Ingredients:
1/2 cup mixed berries (strawberries, blueberries, or raspberries)
1/2 cup low-fat cottage cheese

Preparation:
Combine mixed berries with cottage cheese in a bowl.
Nutritional Information (Approx):
Calories: 120
Protein: 10g
Sodium: 300mg
Potassium: 150mg

1. Berry Blast Smoothie:
Ingredients:
1/2 cup mixed berries (strawberries, blueberries, raspberries)
1/2 banana
1/2 cup low-fat Greek yogurt
1/2 cup water or almond milk (unsweetened)

Preparation:
Blend all ingredients until smooth.
Nutritional Information (Approx):
Calories: 150
Protein: 10g
Sodium: 50mg
Potassium: 200mg

2. Green Spinach and Pineapple Smoothie:
Ingredients:
1 cup fresh spinach leaves
1/2 cup pineapple chunks
1/2 banana
1/2 cup coconut water (unsweetened)

Preparation:
Blend spinach, pineapple, banana, and coconut water until smooth.
Nutritional Information (Approx):
Calories: 120
Protein: 3g
Sodium: 50mg
Potassium: 350mg

3. Creamy Almond Butter Banana Smoothie:
Ingredients:
1 banana
1 tablespoon almond butter
1/2 cup low-fat milk or dairy-free alternative
Ice cubes (optional)

Preparation:
Blend banana, almond butter, milk, and ice cubes
until creamy.
Nutritional Information (Approx):
Calories: 250
Protein: 7g
Sodium: 60mg
Potassium: 300mg

4. Avocado and Berry Protein Smoothie:
Ingredients:
1/4 avocado
1/2 cup mixed berries (strawberries, blueberries,
raspberries)
1/2 cup low-fat Greek yogurt
1/2 cup water or almond milk (unsweetened)

Preparation:
Blend avocado, mixed berries, Greek yogurt, and
water or almond milk until smooth.
Nutritional Information (Approx):
Calories: 180
Protein: 10g
Sodium: 60mg
Potassium: 300mg

5. Tropical Mango and Kiwi Smoothie:
Ingredients:
1/2 cup frozen mango chunks
1 kiwi, peeled and sliced
1/2 cup low-fat coconut milk
1/2 cup water

Preparation:
Blend mango, kiwi, coconut milk, and water until smooth.
Nutritional Information (Approx):
Calories: 160
Protein: 2g
Sodium: 20mg
Potassium: 250mg

Conclusion

In conclusion, the kidney disease food chart serves as a valuable tool for individuals navigating the challenges of managing kidney health through diet. This comprehensive guide provides insights into suitable food choices, portion control, and nutritional considerations tailored to the specific needs of those with kidney disease.

Recognizing the intricate interplay between diet and kidney health, the food chart emphasizes the importance of controlling key nutrients such as sodium, potassium, phosphorus, and protein. These guidelines aim to alleviate the strain on the kidneys, prevent complications, and enhance the overall quality of life for individuals with kidney disease.

The food chart serves as a roadmap for crafting well-balanced meals that support kidney function and help slow the progression of kidney disease. It underscores the significance of individualized nutrition plans, highlighting the unique dietary requirements that vary based on the stage of kidney disease and individual health conditions.

Moreover, the emphasis on collaboration with healthcare professionals and registered dietitians ensures that dietary recommendations align with the specific needs and goals of each individual. Regular consultations and adjustments to the food chart provide a dynamic and responsive approach to managing kidney health through nutrition.

Ultimately, the kidney disease food chart empowers individuals to make informed choices, fostering a proactive role in their well-being. By adhering to these dietary guidelines, individuals can optimize their nutritional intake, control critical elements in their diet, and contribute to the preservation of kidney function.

Incorporating the principles outlined in the kidney disease food chart into daily life not only supports kidney health but also promotes a holistic approach to overall wellness. It is a valuable resource that encourages a mindful and purposeful approach to nutrition, ultimately contributing to an improved quality of life for those navigating the complexities of kidney disease.

My Valued Reader,

I trust this culinary journey has not only ignited your passion for wholesome eating but has also become a haven of inspiration, solace, and invaluable insights. Each carefully curated recipe within this Kidney disease food chart reflects a dedication to excellence, with a profound understanding of the comprehensive guide to the renal diet food list.

Crafted with meticulous attention to detail, these recipes go beyond the realm of mere sustenance; they are a testament to the art of nourishing the body and soul. Your reviews, experiences, and insights are treasures that guide me on this culinary odyssey.

Every evaluation is a stepping stone for refinement, as I aspire to tailor this food chart to surpass your expectations. Let's engage in a dialogue that transcends the pages, creating a connection that resonates with your culinary preferences and well-being goals.

Warm Culinary Regards,

Tina Feldman

www.ingramcontent.com/pod-product-compliance
Lightning Source LLC
Chambersburg PA
CBHW070816260726
48660CB00005B/1870